The Health Effects of Computer Use on Women:

What Every Woman Needs to Know

I0439968

By

Adetutu Ijose

Published By:

Jointheirs Publishing

JP

The Health Effects of Computer Use on
Women:
What Every Woman Needs to Know

Jointheirs Publishing
Jointheirs Activities Incorporated
www.jointheirspublishing.com

ISBN – 1484880145

EAN – 978-1484880142

Printed in the United States of America

The Health Effects of Computer Use on Women:

What Every Woman Needs to Know

An Important Caution

This book is light so do receive it. It is a very great honour for me as a woman, to have been use by our maker to provide this light to women.

The advice given in *The Health Effects of Computer Use on Women* is based on an understanding of the effects of computer use on human health and behavior gained when I a woman, suffered life threatening consequences of computer use that could not be effectively diagnosed or treated by conventional medical science.

I was only able to get an understanding of the problem and identify the solution by studying and gaining an understanding of the human code of existence from studying the System of Nature and human machine user manual we call the Bible or Scriptures. My finding is what is presented in this book.

As in all my other books, I urge the reader to read the entire book and study it carefully.

It is essential that any decision you make be discussed with your physician and parents if you are a not yet an adult or any other person of authority in your life before proceeding.

This book is not meant to replace the advice of parents or the service of a health care provider who knows you personally.

An essential element of taking responsibility for your life and health is a regular medical checkup working in partnership with medical professionals.

If you are under treatment for any computer use induced health condition or if you suspect you might need such care, you must discuss any insight you gain from this book with your doctor before starting.

You can be a long-term computer user without self-destroying but you must first acknowledge the need to do something.

All the solutions are natural, cheap and do not involve medication. In fact medicine is stressful to the body and one that is already weakened from the health effects of computer use should not be medicated. That will increase the stress and start a new problems involving unnecessary costs that could bankrupt individuals and societally as a nation and even globally.

We therefore need to change the way we have been looking at this issue if we want to remain a healthy prosperous population on earth.

One thing though, you must not self diagnose just look for a doctor who is ready to use other measures apart from medication as you will need close monitoring and some tests to identify what is depleted or missing in your body's system as a result of your computer use. These tests do not show everything but are a good starting point.

Computers are here to stay and can never be as safe as claimed. The computer use environment for example makes us look directly at a source of light to read, which is contrary to our natural way of never looking directly at the sun (our natural source of reading light).

Table of Contents

Chapter 1
Introduction to Computer Use

Computers have become indispensable to today's work, study and home environments. Consequently, we are constantly bombarded by it and the access to continuous information.

The quest for knowledge has a partner in the activity of the network of computers we call the Internet.

While access to information is a good thing, there is a saying that too much of anything is bad and that moderation in everything is good.

There is no moderation in today's use of computer systems. This includes access to and use of computer laptops, desktops, tablets such as ipad, cell phones, iphones, video games and so on.

The use of computers has gone beyond information gathering and analysis to leisure, relationships and so on, so that there are now virtual families and home and work/life experiences, meaning that people do not have to live in the real world if they choose to.

They can just keep hooked unto the Internet all day and immerse themselves in a software written by someone to enable the user create the kind of world they like and fantasize all day.

The obvious consequence of this is the high level of strange mental and physiological issues that plague the people in today's world that the medical profession can neither diagnose nor treat.

There is an increasing incidence of people losing their livelihood and even their lives due to medical issues arising from computer use.

While there are many issues that affect all computer users, there are also issues unique to men and some unique to women

These issues are mainly based on the hormonal differences between the genders and the different manifestations of the susceptibility to the health effect of an activity such as computer use as a result of these hormonal differences.

There is a general acknowledgement for example, of a higher cancer episode in women computer operators than in men.

Women also seem to have more of the emotional issues such as feeling they are not getting cooperation from others on the job and feeling that they are constantly being misunderstood.

In chapters 3 to 8, I discuss the reasons for these issues and the gender differences that are responsible for them.

Life and light

Life is light and the life light in us helps us to handle various natural light fields because we are coded with them and mechanisms are in us to handle them unless for example we are struck by a bolt of lightning, an overdose of natural electrical current beyond which the human body has the capability to handle.

The problem in today's world is that we are constantly exposed to artificial lights that have no life and are not the same configuration as the natural ones.

For it is impossible for anyone to develop natural light.

The code is in the word in the mouth of our creator. Hence we do not have access to and can never have access to it and since light cannot be seen or touched we can only guess at its composition we do not know it.

Therefore, experimenting as we are constantly doing instead of believing the word of our code, which he has mercifully provided to us we are finding, is foolhardy and self destructive.

Yet humanity seem to be unable to get off the course of self destruction it has embarked upon and everyone has become schizophrenic running away from our maker instead of running to him for repair.

Women used to be the voice of reason, the ones to hold everybody accountable, now women vie to be more destructive than men if possible.

This is evidence of the fact that all we have been doing has been weakening our light fields so we are not able to operate properly as coded, afraid of the truth and unwilling to repent yet seeking forgiveness the condition for which is repentance.

All our experiments are only trial and error guesswork, which is why our science is always changing because we are not operating in the realm of the maker just as the computer is not operating in our realm.

We are coded beings, meaning we are limited to the flexibilities provided in our code for effective functioning. When we go beyond that as we currently are, we become malfunctioning computers full of viruses, malware, worms and so on.

This is the reason we have all these computer use induced health problems.

Computer use violates our coded way of being and operating as humans. Though our maker knowing we would come to this point placed systems and tools in nature to help us, we have shut him out and refused to acknowledge we are out of whack.

Many of us are not fully aware there is a problem and only acknowledge it when it is far gone.

We are exposed to what our bodies are not coded for.

However, the computer is a dangerous tool just like the knife.

And just as we had to learn how to use the knife so as not to hurt ourselves so we have to do with the computer especially as we have made our lives to revolve around it.

Overly wired.
In today's world everyone is overly wired from office computers to apps to call phones and many spend their leisure time on faccebook and other social websites instead of getting some sunlight to boost their biochemical resource levels.

This has huge health and mental consequences as our systems become overloaded and we find both home and work chores a huge burden.

We never have time, because computer use addiction is epidemic globally today.

In some cases it is what people's careers demand. However instead of limiting outside office computer use, many such people spend as much if not more time outside office work browsing the Internet, gaming and on social websites as well as reading and sending emails.

The computer, instead of they controlling it, controls them.

Many a times errors are made at work because we are trying to multitask – work and use the phone at the same time.

As women and mothers and wives who are responsible for providing a moral compass for others, as we read this book, I urge us to be truthful with ourselves and make the required changes to enable us to be that compass that we were created to be for our homes.

Chapter 2
Light

Light is the basis for life. It is the light of life that powers humans and everything else in nature.

Light comes in various levels of intensity and purity

The human is three dimensional – spirit, soul and body.

Each of these dimensions has its light fields. For light from one dimension to operate in another dimension, it passes on its message to the light in that dimension.

The light in a particular dimension controls that dimension and all dimensions lower than it. Hence the light in the spirit dimension is above that of the soul and the physical.

For it to operate in the physical the corresponding light in the soul dimension and the physical that is required for the action to be taken in the physical must be present.

The spirit would pass the message to the soul and the soul to the physical. It needs the light in both the soul and the physical dimension to operate in the physical dimension.

The user manual given to us by our maker we call the Bible or Scriptures tells us that when the earth was created, it was, not discernable and was covered with darkness and had no inhabitants until the maker introduced light into the environment of nature in which the earth was created.

This was what gave rise to day and night. Prior to that, time did not exist it was all darkness and endless night i.e. an eternity of night. There was no time period. It was one endless night until nature was ready to be revealed at which point light was introduced to reveal it and give it life.

When light was introduced it obliterated all darkness and brought about a new kind of eternity, endless day.

The manual tells us our maker found the light to be very good. This would be the end of the code i.e. the end product, a creation that would be in endless day i.e. light where there is no darkness, just like the maker.

There however needed to be a process to take the creation from being in endless night to endless day.

There needed to be a period of co habitation of day and night so that the inhabitants of this creation could be brought forth and gradually refined to become light where there is no darkness at all able to handle eternal light and life and day.

Light was introduced and made to co exist with darkness creating day and night. This was created to provide a time of rest away from the direct glare of the light in order to enable the bodies of matter to self repair and refine.

This environment of day and night i.e. of light and darkness is the environment into which humans and all other living beings on earth were placed when they were made and given life to dwell here on the earth where they would be refined along with the earth from which they are made.

They would be the barometer that would reflect how refined the earth was and how much more refinement is required to enable the earth be strong enough to handle and become eternal light.

In this period of refinement, the daytime is for activity and the nighttime for rest and repair.

Illumination

Light is what reveals what is around. The light in a particular realm exposes the things in that realm that the intensity of light in that realm can reveal.

There could be things in a realm that are unseen in that realm but which may be visible in a different realm that contains the kind of light that can expose the kind of material whether darkness or some other matter not available in the physical realm we humans live in.

The physical body as the user manual tells us has no life of its own but is managed, operated and powered by light fields we call biochemicals. The light fields connect the soul to the physical.

The soul receives light from the spirit that it passes to the body for action.

As we read in chapter 1, the code of our being is written in light, which we cannot see nor have access to.

We only see the result of the operating code. The biochemicals we call neurotransmitters are the messaging light fields that pass the instruction of our code to the various parts of the body for action.

The realm of the biochemicals is the soul realm, which is why attempts to medicate it never really works for there is no medicine that can produce light fields of life.

The soul lights called biochemicals pass life from the spirit to the physical body empowering it to move and talk and run and so on.

What we can do, our emotions and activities are dependent on the balance and quantity of these fields we have in our bodies.

If we fail to carry out an action we need to ,it is because we either have insufficient amount of the messaging light required or they are missing.

Indeed word is light but word in different realms is different dimensions of light operating in the different realms and only revealing things in the realms in which they operate.

Our user manual actually tells us that everything was created and brought into being by word.

The messaging light fields that operate us are word light fields. They speak and convey the messaging words of our code and empower the various parts of our being to operate by the word of command they speak.

The human machine vs. the computer
As the human machine is three dimensional, computers and other objects fashioned after it that have motion and activity are also 3 dimensional.

To recap, the human is made up of the physical body that the manual tells us on its own has no life. Science tells us we have about five billion cells. In fact our body cells do not speak to each other and cannot operate on their own but they are as we have read in this chapter, operated, given life and direction by what we call biochemicals.

If we have never heard of biochemcals these are things such as enzymes, hormones such as estrogen and progesterone, neurotransmitters such as Gamma-amino butyric acid (GABA), serotonin, dopamine, noradrenalin and so on that operate, maintain and repair the whole human body machine system.

They pass nutrients through the blood into every cell giving it life Hence the physical we can see and touch is operated by that we cannot see or touch this is the soul realm where the biochemicals reside.

Biochemicals cannot be seen or touched for they are light fields that act like chemicals. Where do they come from? The light that powers us comes from the sun, moon and stars especially the sun. These are the only light we are coded with by our maker who also has coded life into us through this light.

It is the life in the light that converts the light (electromagnetic fields) we receive into that which can operate in us and all other living beings that operate on the earth such as animals, insects and plants.

That is why we can eat them and obtain life fields and biochemicals such as enzymes, hormones pre formed neurotransmitters, amino acids and so on from them. Indeed all living things on the earth all have the same biochemicals. The soul level where the biochemicals reside, operates the body.

The third dimension is the spirit of life that gives life to the soul and that comes directly and is totally under the direct control of our maker alone.

For the computer, the three dimensions are – the physical computer device is the first dimension. The second is the artificially generated electromagnetic fields of lifeless light that projects the words and images we see on the screen and operates the system and the third is the raw artificially generated lifeless electrical electromagnetic field that comes from the power plant.

So for the body we have light from the sun moon and stars that have life. That light is broken down and used to produce new light or electromagnetic field fields in us called biochemicals that have life and these then produce life activities such as eating, sleeping, walking, thinking and so on in us.

The computer has lifeless light from the power plant that produces lifeless electromagnetic field in the computer when passed through certain magnetic fields and these light fields are used to project lifeless pictures and words and other images unto lifeless computer screens for us to see.

Hence though we are only coded with light that has life computer use brings us in contact with lifeless light, which is harmful or toxic to our souls that are coded to only be in the presence of light that has life. We will see the effect this has next.

It is like putting software that a computer system is not coded to handle into it. It may operate well for some time and seem to cope because of the built in repair system but it will eventually crash. That is what we call sickness and diseases.

Statics

One of the strange conditions that afflicted me as a result of computer use was statics coming off from my palms anytime I touched anything even paper or plastic. It was very weird. I could not touch anything without statics coming off.

In addition, some oil came off my hands and soiled everything I touched. It was scary

This only got resolved after I started working on naturally building up my inhibitory neurotransmitters through diet, exercise and sun therapy. I will discuss many of these solutions throughout this book.

I will also recommend that anyone wanting to know more should read my other books. There are 14 of them as at the time of the writing of this book and a list is provided in the "Note to the Reader"

Computer Vision Syndrome and Light Sensitivity

As a cumulative effect of constant bombardment of computer light from long hours in front of a computer without adequate breaks to expose the body to natural light, a woman's system could become overcharged with toxic electrical current from the computer as well as indoor lighting.

I suffered this and had to take time off away from all unnatural light in addition to diet and exercise with reading with the light of the sun daily to detoxify.

If we are so glued to technology products that we have more of artificial than natural light fields in our system we could actually collapse.

Some women have told me stories of their husbands dying from this because no one could diagnose what the problem was.

The truth is that the issue of computer use induced health conditions is not well known in the medical profession that is totally geared towards solving everything with medication.

When it is confronted with something that cannot be medicated, it is unable to provide a diagnosis or solution.

In such instances, people are misdiagnosed as the more commonly known ailment closest to it and medicated with dire consequences that are also misdiagnosed creating a cycle of ever changing drugs and ailments.

The consequence of this, is that the initial problem is not resolved while new ones are introduced as a result of the misdiagnosis.

Many doctors are yet to admit that computer use can hurt and tell patients "it is all in your mind" because these issues cannot be diagnosed or effectively detected by man made diagnostic tools.

In addition, because sufferers find it difficult to actually describe what they are feeling due to messaging biochemical deficiency misdiagnosis is routine.

Yet the medical profession is critical to the process as computer use induced health conditions are serious and sufferers need close monitoring.

The purpose of this and all my other books is to give computer users a tool that helps them understand and have words to verbalize their ailments.

It is important that a physician be consulted who is willing to use non medication based treatment.

In fact it is dangerous to self diagnose computer use induced health conditions.

My advise is that you get books that are relevant to your issue to your doctor and discuss with him or her because you need to be monitored if you are trying to reverse an issue.

It may also help if readers spread the information about my books to everyone.

I believe if most people know about these books and begin to understand themselves, pressure can be brought to bear upon the medical profession to change.

Far too much money is being wasted by people on unnecessary or even counter productive treatment and care.

As I will discuss in this book and as I have in my other books, the solutions to computer use induced health conditions are in most cases free and not onerous.

The only thing is that it must be carried out consistently whether we feel like it or not. Do not be fooled by your feelings. They can be very deceptive.

The human machine user manual we call the Bible or Scriptures expressly tells us not to allow our feeling to dictate to us, but the code as presented to us in the manual should determine our actions ensuring our system operate according to the code of our being.

The code of our being

The manual tells us that the code of nature started with an earth encased in water and as we read earlier in this chapter, surrounded with darkness that was not discernable and did not have the kind of landscape we have today.

It was an eternity of darkness when time was non existent.

Then light was introduced to create day and night and provide an opportunity to refine nature.

The coded process will end with an eternal day just as it started with an eternal night.

Consequently, it is going from one eternity to another. Time is the process in between the two eternities to refine nature and all that therein is for the eternal day.

In a coded system, everything that needs to take place to arrive at the end must be pre planned and coded in as the manual tells us it was, and controls and events for self correction must also be put in place.

Consequently, all the happenings we are seeing today is not chaos but part of the process of refinement and self correction put in place by our maker.

It is the only way to go from an eternity of darkness to an eternity of light.

Our maker has however given all his works a freewill to chose whether to be part of the eternity of light or not. For only light can be in an eternity of light.

Objects we see today are essentially solid darkness. For an object in the physical realm is formed from solid darkness emitting light in such a fashion as to create each kind of object.

Anything that does not emit light cannot be seen. It will exist in darkness but will not be seen because darkness needs light to reveal what is in it.

Luminous bodies have an abundance of light and go beyond emitting to radiating and transmitting light in such a high voltage that they can provide light to other beings that can ignite the low levels of light in them and make them to emit light and be seen, move around and so on.

This light that they transmit is what we receive as neurotransmitters, which are converted in us, as we will discuss later in this book, to the form in which it can operate in us.

Light is comfortable but darkness is not

Darkness is the absence of light and is the exact opposite of light. Hence darkness is the reversal of the code of created light.

There is physical darkness and spiritual darkness just as there is physical light and spiritual light.

Darkness and thoughts that originate from it is not comfortable though humans like to self deceive that it is okay. After some time of self deception one would question it.

However the human heart, which is the physical central command of the body that controls the physical body matter in its analysis is able to come up with rationalization that gets changed routinely to fit whatever is being proposed out of darkness. More on this later in the book.

Light, Pigmentation and iron

The amount of light we can receive and retain as humans depends on the amount of pigmentation we have.

While women are more likely to have depression than men, it is also commonly known that there is more occurrence of mental issues and depression in people with less pigmentation.

Because of this issue, though everyone needs to ensure they have daily access to sunlight, people with European lineage must make double sure they do so especially in today's computer use dependent world to ensure they can handle life's stresses.

A mineral that is heavily used in light absorption is iron.

It used to be common knowledge that people of European descent were generally never iron deficient but in today's world that is changing and many are finding themselves becoming iron deficient without knowing why.

It is because iron is heavily used in receiving the computer light that is transmitted to us including the images and words we receive. Meanwhile nobody eats to meet the nutritional requirements for computer use.

.

Chapter 3
The Virtual World, Video Games and so on

Humans were conditioned and prepared themselves for the virtual world when movies, television and videos came into being.

Women gobbled it up as it enabled them temporarily escape the myriad of real and imagined problems they had in their lives.

While men love watching sports, news, politics i.e. real life happenings. Women love the make belief. They love to see enacted their imagination before their eyes rather than the reality.

This may have been what led the first woman into the first mistake. She had big plans for her husband and was ready to believe the lie because it fed into her wondering mind and imagination of what if?

The same biochemicals that were deficient then are still the same ones needed today

Aversion for truth
A consequence of our having watched so many movies and television and read so many gossip columns, novels and other fiction is that it makes lying so easy and creates an aversion for truth unless it is something pleasant according to our heart, which is where all words and images and thoughts are received.

Computer use makes us depleted in critical light fields of biochemicals necessary to handle stress and discern truth as they are used up by the activity of computer use without being replenished because they can only be replenished from life containing light from the sun, moon and stars.

This is probably the reason why many are ready to take risks while on the Internet and are so easily led into dangerous online relationships.

Many people are careless when chatting and write things they would never say in person as comments on blogs and social media websites.

Virtual (artificial/imaginary) Lives

There are now many websites where one can basically live a virtual life of imagination with just the right spouse and children and job, bosses and so on so that life is perfect.

This can be dangerous making it difficult for people to have real life relationships as they try to transfer their virtual lives into reality or become recluse living for the Internet.

This kind of Internet activity could take over a person's life. Getting access to and living at this websites is not cheap and can lead to the same issues as gambling once people become dependent on it.

There is even virtual (artificial) sex, kissing and so on. This would have sounded bizarre before the advent of the computer when people started losing their ability to correctly discern what is right and wrong and lost their sense of discretion and shame.

Now there is nothing to be ashamed of and everything right or wrong is okay.

When the repercussions of these acts come such as broken homes, broken real relationships, loss of finance, businesses, jobs and so on people sometimes still are unable to face reality and feel they have been badly treated.

This is the result of the depletion in biochemical light fields.

The user manual given to us by our maker actually tells us the thoughts of our hearts, which most of us base our actions on cannot be relied upon.

As the manual says we all need to read the human machine user manual more and use it as our basis of action. We should weigh whatever we are doing by it and ask ourselves if we want the repercussion it tells us will come our way before acting

As we have read in this book, the manual actually tells us not to be led by the thoughts of our hearts but by the code of our being presented to us in the manual.

I have discovered that it has an answer for everything and that following it ensures that our human system work as intended.

Video games

In every area women compete with men for pre eminence including in owning video games.

We are just as wired as the men and many of us are getting our children wired at an early age when their brains are still developing.

This issue of exposing our children to all these "absent yet being present" way of life as a result of being continually wired may require rethinking and active corrective work.

If we are overly wired we will neither have the capability nor moral authority to keep our children in line, with horrible consequences for the future.

These children did not beg to come here. We brought them here and are responsible for giving them at least the level of guidance we got when we were growing up and even more because of the horrible issues they have to deal with in their generation.

It is foolhardy to compete with men on what we have hormonal disadvantages for and that results in harm.

What is the point in trying to be the gender that can self destroy the most.

When we find out things are not as rosy as we would want them to be, we try to fake things, forgetting that we thereby lure other women to make the same mistake we regret, when we pretend in order to be thought of as being tough..

The nature and human machine user manual says we will have to account for every soul we mislead.

For more information on this subject please refer to my book – *The Health Effects of Video Games.*

Chapter 4
The female hormonal balance

Women because of their delicate hormonal balance especially the estrogen/progesterone balance needs may find themselves feeling overly stressed by long hours of computer use

Women grow up needing a balance in their estrogen to progesterone levels for a sense of wellbeing especially after they reach puberty.

When this balance is off, the resultant stress to the female system can be expressed by the body in the form of mood swings, depression, cancer and a host of other issues.

Consequently, any environment that has a potential of affecting this delicate balance is a recipe for all kinds of health and relationship issues.

There is a part of the artificial light that comes off the computer screen that mimics the biochemical light field or hormone called estrogen.

This, as well as toxic artificially generated chemicals and minerals, such as silicon, used in making computer monitor screens, keyboards, cables and other computer parts, that both front end and back end computer users and operators come in contact with, can affect this delicate balance.

For women in the pre menopausal, menopausal or postmenopausal stages when natural estrogen production reduces, the body may replace its shortfall with this toxic estrogen.

Artificial estrogen or estrogen like chemicals that reflect off the computer screen could actually derail the balance in a toxic way in women of all ages, as the body finds it difficult or virtually impossible to use this estrogen that could become more abundant than natural estrogen in the body creating all kinds of havoc in the system that no drug can arrest.

When this happens the only recourse is to detoxify and avoid computer light exposure.

In today's world this solution is virtually impossible to implement, as computers have become indispensable to our way of living.

Since avoidance may be difficult, women may need to consider avoiding other avoidable sources of artificial estrogen and other stress causing artificial chemicals and light such as non organic/Genetically Modified (GMO) foods, poorly ventilated environments, household chemical sprays, artificial chemical containing cosmetic product and so on to prevent the body from being overwhelmed by toxins,

An added problem is the abundance of soy a highly estrogenic food whose estrogen the body finds difficult to digest in our foods. Virtually everything has soy added to it in one way or another.

Many computer users are guilty of eating an abundance of processed food, as it is easy to grab and eat, to satisfy the hunger pangs that come with excessive computer use, which most people are guilty of.

The need for rebalancing cannot be over emphasized.

How can we rebalance? Here are a few suggestions, more will be provided in other chapters of this book.

Some simple rebalancing activities include going for long walks during the day (take time to look at the green grass, leaves and other natural beauties, crack open the window to allow natural rebalancing of inside air, read with the light of the sun daily (especially the human computer user manual we call the Bible to get a better understanding of the human body's code of existence).

Eat plenty of organic fruits and vegetables as well as whole grains. Cook at home more often to get a better control of what you are actually eating.

Take many breaks while working and make an effort to blink often, have daily positive inter personal physical face to face conversation and contact with others especially family members (avoid negative issues.

 Learn to say sorry quickly and do not insist on always being right. Talk less and listen more), help someone in need as often as possible in easy simple ways and so on.

Sense of wellbeing and discernment

The hormonal balance thrown off by the artificial estrogen in computer light coupled with depletions in inhibitory neurotransmitters responsible for the feeling of well being such as serotonin can have very serious consequence on a woman's sense of well being and security

Remember the biochemicals called neurotransmitters we discussed in earlier chapters, the over production of excitatory neurotransmitter leading to depletion in them as well, may affect our ability to exercise caution leading

many to do things such as sexting i.e. texting nude photos
of themselves and so on.
For more information on this issue please refer to my book
– *Teenage and Ault texting addictions*

It may even lead some to put their child in danger without
realizing it. There are mothers who feel so overwhelmed
they give their ipads to babies whose brains are still
developing.

This issue may be why so many women are now losing
their ability to even understand themselves as women and
decide to go for sex change or leave their homes in search
of some feelings that they feel they are not getting from
their husbands and homes.

Self control and Sexual Adventurism

As we read in earlier chapters, biochemical light field
depletions inherent in computer use make people less risk
averse.

This has become worrisome in issues such as faithfulness
in marriage.

The manual tells us the man is corrected by the behavior of
his wife. This is where the first woman failed her husband
she did not humble herself and was too ready to believe
what her imagination was telling her

In today's world, the men are no longer checked when it
comes to fidelity by the behavior of their wives

The stories of women cheating on their husbands and
feeling cool about it until everything goes wrong is on the
rise.

I will now touch a sensitive area.

Everyone is born male or female. It is impossible to be born both. The sexual organs are connected to the urinary/bladder system and only one can be connected in each person.

As we read in chapter 2, the human system and indeed the whole of nature is a coded system. The manual provides us with the beginning and the end of the code, showing us what the desired end product is, as well as everything that has been put in nature as controls to ensure the desired end is achieved.

Consequently, when people feel they should be a different sex from that in which they were born it is not physiological. It is only in their thoughts.

We are not born with our thoughts but thoughts are a matter of what the heart chooses to receive based on what we have seen and heard since we were born.

Many would want to blame their inability to change their thought process on their birth but that is wishful thinking and not truth.

The popular belief these days of being born this way is fallacy and does not agree with the way coded beings are made.

The lack of understanding or appreciation of the fact that we are coded being and the implication of that is why this narration has taken root in addition to fear because we heterosexuals too are not handling things right.

We heterosexuals should learn from Lot and Abraham in the manual. God has given everyone a free will to choose.

When people make wrong choices as fundamental as that of homosexuality, they need help and encouragement to get them to go though the most likely very difficult process of repentance.

The people that have done this publicly and who have given their account and even written books about their experience say it entailed a very hard process. This indicates that these people who make these wrong decisions need all the encouragement we can give them.

Like Lot, we should tell them what they are doing is wrong but not take the grace of God from them for who knows whether that person will be willing to change.

We are responsible for showing them by the way we conduct ourselves the beauty and blessedness of operating the right way.

Abraham did not refuse to save the homosexuals in Sodom when they were taken captive, but rescued the whole of Sodom when he went to rescue his nephew Lot when the whole town was taken captive.

Our maker also provides us with an example of how to relate to these people. He allowed them to be prosperous. In fact everything was made easy for them though they did not repent. That was their choice.

They were given a long time, and when the earth had enough of the darkness they were producing as a result of not operating according to the human coded way of operation, it rejected them. God in his mercy still gave a final chance because he does not want any to be destroyed but repentance is what he wants.

They however brought their own destruction upon themselves as they refused to repent and nature was in the self repair mode, removing anything producing excessive darkness as sexual activity contrary to the code does.

It makes the body be a human computer that cannot produce holy seed from sexual activity, which the manual tells us such activity is primarily for.

Anything that foments darkness will be thrown out of nature sooner or later because as we said in chapter 2, the process is running a code that started in eternal darkness and which is going to an end of eternal light.

Consequently, anything that is not progressing towards eternal light will be removed in due course.

It is also obvious that in the European pagan/occult culture of old, homosexuality was an acceptable practice, which people tried to stop when the light of Christianity came around and people realized it could never be acceptable to our maker.

However artificial Christianity, which is a merger of Christianity with European occult practice and outright presumptuous false doctrine not taught by Paul or found anywhere in Scriptures was what took hold.

This is what has been spread all over the earth. My advise is - stick to what the Bible says. Read it yourself.

Consequently, for some people, the high level occult practice, which must be in place for one to lose the fundamental light fields that must be lost before homosexuality can take place, is what they have received as tradition from their ancestors.

If true Christianity had been adopted in European instead of the merger with the occult, this issue would probably not be around today. Unfortunately, the European Occult practice has been spread round the world with the spread of homosexuality as part of the consequence, as others have been brought into the occult and afflicted too.

Now we have a global problem.

More Explanation

Our ability to analyze things properly and take the right decisions is dependent on the balance of neurotransmitters in us.

We can only carry out the actions we have neurotransmitters to pass the necessary code of instructions for actions on.

Since neurotransmitters are light fields it means the ability of our hearts to effectively use our brains to correctly analyze thoughts we receive depends on the light fields of words stored in the database of our hearts and the availability of messaging light fields or messaging words of instruction/commands necessary to select the right words from our database.

After correct analysis, there is also the question off the availability of light fields of command to carry out the necessary instructions.

Any depletion in any of these steps will lead to wrong action.

This is why many say they struggle with such thoughts as homosexuality and are unable to control themselves.

It is because along the way they have carried out some actions that resulted in their losing the light fields that would have in the first place protected them from such thoughts (nobody is born with the thoughts of their hearts. Thoughts are a user defined activity that involves the activity of the soul and the heart operating in this physical realm)

They have also lost or have become depleted in the ones that would enable them reject such thoughts or they were careless and not vigilant or deceived themselves or listened to deceptive words of others (written in books, magazine or spoken in the media or directly to them) that it was a good idea to experiment and did not consider a one time action a threat just to find out what it is like.

All these are indication of the loss of protective light fields we are born with.

Because sexual orientation is fundamental to who we are - the manual tell us that humans were made to be distinctly male or female and the physical sexual organs in each body is what determines that.

Our maker has given us a freewill to choose our thoughts and consequently our actions.

All thoughts are external as we discussed earlier in this book and come from the celestial realms that are above the earth including from satellites and other man made entities in outer space being used to conduct manipulative experiments at the expense of the whole human race.

To lose our ability to act as our physical body dictates is evidence of a serious shortfall in the messaging system in place to empower our organs to automatically ac the way they are constructed to.

It means an override of the original has happened.
That tells you there is a way to override the normal code of operation for actions controlled by thoughts. The thoughts we choose can override and create action contrary to the norm.

As we have read in this chapter, for the fundamental kind of override involved in homosexuality, something drastic must have happened to make the messaging neurotransmitter group to become so depleted that it malfunctions.

It takes very contrary thought choices and actions to make the light to recede to that level because the manual tells us the purpose of bringing men and women together i.e. the purpose for having two sexes is for the purpose of child bearing.

It means our sexual organs are coded in a way to carry only actions that would result in creating babies, which we are told is the purpose of sex.

Consequently, it would take a dark action somewhere for this fundamental purpose to be overridden.

Hence without occult practice by a person e.g., Lodges, Fraternities, Sororities, Wicca, Sorceries of all sorts, witchcraft, Metaphysics, Yoga meditation and so on there can be no homosexuality.

The light of normal female activity must recede and it will only recede with a decision by a person to do something so obnoxious to light that it decides it does not want to preserve that soul and body again.

For when the right orientation is lost, that person has lost their purpose for being.

They are unable to bring forth children and teach them in the way of our maker.

What homosexuality really means is a disagreement with the maker's purpose.

The work around of just having children outside of normal heterosexual relationships and using sperm donors, surrogates and so on will not work (you cannot bribe the maker. The rules are cast in stone. It will not count as bringing forth seed).

The manual tells us our maker wants us to be obedient. He said "obedience is better than sacrifice".

I have taken time to explain all this to help people to understand themselves and others so they do not wander into things and wonder how they got there.

Occult activity must be somewhere either carried out by the person themselves or their parents etc. Many do not want to acknowledge and maybe do not realize that the consequence of joining occult groups can be felt generations down.

In addition, there is no free lunch in the occult even if you are promised one. You automatically lose light fields when you go into the cult and leave yourself open to a lot of dark thoughts.

That is why it is said that the only solution to homosexuality is through turning to our maker. He must recreate those light field if they are totally lost and if depleted he must provide the enablement and conducive environment to rebuild the abundance of light fields again.

Computer use depletions would make it difficult for people who want to turn around from doing so unless they make an effort to build up their light field with activities such as prayer, Bible reading, and departure from any activity that is not righteous.

They may have to change their job to that which will not require them to lie or do anything that increases the darkness in them.

The Pineal Gland

Another thing to consider is the imagination of humans. As we read in chapter 2, light is received in informational form in 2 ways, images and words.

The pineal gland in the inner part of the brain is what the heart uses for imaginary analysis of thoughts it receives. It runs it like a video or film. This is the basis of our understanding of how to make movies and videos

It is the part of the brain that is tampered with by occult practice to get the so called "third eye" and it is when it is tampered with that people can see into the spiritual part of the occult realm.

The normal function of this gland is for receiving visions and dreams from our maker. It also plays a role in sexual activity because of the part that the imagination takes in sexual activity.

When this area is tampered with people have fake/false/artificial dreams and all kinds of occult attacks and hear voices and see all kinds or horrible terrible things.

It can be used to torment people and affect their reasoning. The messaging system that affects this gland the most is melatonin, a neurotransmitter that is also a hormone, which is produced at night when the sun goes down.

Constantly being on the computer late at night could affect the rhythm of its production.

Taking melatonin supplements to restore melatonin levels can help if done in conjunction with attempts to restore the rhythm by sleeping early and waking up with the sun, getting adequate sunlight exposure, GABA supplementation, with diet and exercise.

As with all other neurotransmitter there is not just one type of melatonin. That is why it takes a multi pronged approach to built up depletion in any neurotransmitter.

They also work in groups. Consequently, trying to build up one, needs the building up of several others i.e. the main depletion and the secondary ones.

I am writing this because it seems to me that the number of people becoming homosexuals is on the rise and I am seeking to help people know the truth about what is happening to them.

What I have written is what the maker has revealed to me to write because I kept on seeing so many reports of people becoming homosexuals and being deceived that somehow God was responsible for their predicament and that it was acceptable to him.

I also noticed that even some Christian Churches were deceiving people and telling them it was a blessing – giving people false hopes, lying against God and the Scriptures thereby taking away the grace of God from these people. After praying for understanding on why humans can go so off code, it was explained to me so I could write it in this book and any of my other books where I have touched this subject.

One does not need to experience this issue to understand it. One only needs to understand that humans are coded beings and understand the code of the human machine.

Melatonin levels and early access to computers

Since people are now getting access to the computer at a very young age, instead of their melatonin levels being high as it should be to balance the high adrenalin and other excitatory neurotransmitter levels, thereby protecting them, it is low and girls and boys too are reaching puberty and becoming aware of themselves sexually earlier than they should.

This opens them up to dark thoughts they may not be able to handle without parental guidance if their parents are involved in any kind of occult activity.

Many parents do not realize that occult activity brings the practitioner and their family into the line of attack. Many do not realize that some of the oaths they make is an open door to their family members.

When the repercussion comes few if any are willing to tell the truth about their involvement in the occult.

Young women who get into lodges, sororities and yoga and other occult activities may find themselves experiencing more negative sexual tendencies and wanting adventure, unable to really weigh the risk and just falling into whatever comes along because their light levels are low.

Bottom line

So how should we relate to the homosexual. Like Lot and Abraham did. Tell them the truth and leave them to make their choice. Everyone is entitled to their choice and no one can force anyone to make a right choice.

We should tell the truth about sororities, lodges, fraternities and other occult groups and the connection between the occult and homosexuality.

We should also get a copy of this book to them so they understand the extent of their vulnerabilities and the truth.

We should provide a conducive environment for them to be able to change and repent if they choose to, like God did for the people of Sodom and Gomorrah, They had everything but the manual tells us they were wicked.

They took the maker's benevolence for granted and refused to listen to Lot.

Thus the manual classifies unwillingness to change from homosexuality as wickedness but allows people to chose it if they want while leaving an open door for repentance.

It is not sugarcoated in the manual. We are told that homosexuality is an abomination to God. Since God calls it an abomination, that is what it is and nobody can change it.

We are however in the period of grace before nature fully self corrects removing everything that cannot proceed to be fully light.
Heterosexuals, committing adultery, pedophiles and other sins both sexual and otherwise are all conditions for being removed as part of the correction.

Consequently, let everyone concentrate on their own self correction instead of comparing themselves to others and declaring themselves to be more righteous than they are.

It is only the maker himself that initiates the process of self correction, granting the earth its desire for self correction and removal of darkness it finds intolerable. No human has a right to enforce the self correction of nature and no one can.

We should just do what is right and leave nature to self correct as it will, to avoid being accused of over reaching and being swept away in the correction. That was Lot's attitude and that is what saved him. He spoke and left the people to make their choices.

Everybody has a choice and will ultimately individually bear the consequence of his or her choice. That is a fundamental human right given to each one by our maker who has written the consequence for every action into the code of our being.

The code is continuously running its course from day to day according to what is written in the code of our being.

There are some things that can be reversed and some cannot. For example time cannot be reversed.

If we go beyond our authority we will be swept away too.

This is the period of grace and all are entitled to grace. Like I wrote earlier in this chapter, who knows who will repent. Anyone who tries to prevent another from receiving grace runs the risk of losing grace themselves.

Also remember that the manual tells us anything from darkness must always run its course and reach its peak before full correction takes place to allow for repentance since it is not the maker's will that anyone be destroyed.

He however will let people have their way while leaving room for their salvation if they turn to him
That is why the maker has allowed the changes to the law we have seen here in the USA, to take place so no one has an excuse for their action.

No one can now say it was because they had so much opposition, they were unable to change as they used all their neurotransmitter resources just to stay above all the oppression. That is no longer tenable.

People can also take their choice to the logical conclusion of being completely overtaken by darkness.

According to the manual, because of grace, humans must reach the fullness of their self destruction before nature commences its universal correction. As this issue is now a global one and natural corrective action will also be global.

I believe that there are probably many more homosexuals than people think and the darkness is much more than people assume it is. The fullness of it and all other sins must be exposed before correction can take place as it happened in the days of Noah. It is round the corner.

This all just shows us that nature's self correction is about to take place. It is the code running. Letting everyone have their way so there are no grey areas. Everyone can make a clear choice without any ambiguity, making it easy to effect detoxification of nature.

The truth is that occultism is not compatible with technology and computer use as they both produce an enormous amount of darkness.

Many people want homosexuality to come to an end. Here is how – end all occultism. Take it out of the Church and out of everything else – politics, social life, music, entertainment, academia, education, medicine, science, medicine and so on. I mean out of everything with no exception.

We either do it willingly or it will be done for us in the self corrective process of nature, when the code reaches the process required to eliminates excessive darkness because the bottom line is an earth and nature in eternal day forever.

That is the end product of the code of nature running, which we are a part of.

Chapter 5
The Female emotional balance

Women and men produce the various inhibitory and excitatory neurotransmitters and other biochemicas common to both sexes in varying proportions.

The result of this is the existence of two kinds of humans male and female.

Because the maker made the man for procreation but did not make him to be able to do that by himself, without help, women were created to be help meet to men in bringing forth children.

They had to have an emotional balance tuned to discerning, interpreting and meeting the needs of dependent infants. They also had to be able to move quickly to avert danger and meet their infant's need for comfort and feeding.

They had to be able to identify the needs of their infant in the midst of others

Consequently, they had to be able to react fast and anticipate the change in an infant's need for food, comfort, protective help from danger or sickness and disease. It meant attention to detail and ability to change course quickly.

Therefore, as women enter the childbearing age, they produce more excitatory neurotransmitters such as adrenalin and less of inhibitory neurotransmitters that inhibit production of excitatory ones.

Consequently, women are not generally as calm as men and fly off the handle more easily.

This has implications for mental health issues such as depression that is a result of inadequate production of inhibitory neurotransmitters.

Because women naturally produce a high level of excitatory neurotransmitters, anything that depletes the availability of inhibitors with consequent production of yet more excitatory neurotransmitters will create an imbalance.

This is the reason for the varying levels of depression between men and women in the general population on the earth. Women are more inclined to suffer depression than men.

Since computer use results in the depletion of inhibitors it is obvious that the mental health effect of computer use will generally be felt a lot more by women.

That is why we feel the workplace burnout more and find that we are more feelings oriented.

We feel more easily overwhelmed because it is the inhibitors such as GABA that enable us handle the stress of life and keep us calm.

It is this imbalance that makes us very reactionary. We react to everything and are more quick to call it quits when our feelings are offended, feel that others are not cooperating and so on.

Notice it is the feelings not necessarily the facts of the situation. That is because the balance of neurotransmitters in us, control our feelings.

The man on the other hand is not into every detail. He looks at the big picture and leads and protects by being calm. Which is the exact opposite of the woman who protects by reacting and losing control.

Hence we as women are always trying to control because we feel a sense of danger and lack of control.

Men consequently produce more inhibitors naturally. As they grow older they are calmer and less prone to fight.

When they are younger they are more prone to fighting as the neurotransmitters that control the production of testosterone is in abundance.

Though women produce more excitatory neurotransmitters, they are curtailed by the lower muscle mass they have than men.

The lower production in excitatory neurotransmitters in men is compensated by the higher male muscle mass.

Other Issues
Sleep walking
I have seen people who as a result of high electricity exposure because of their jobs find themselves sleepwalking, becoming susceptibility to satellites and other energy sources from space being beamed down for occult reason and experimental satellite activity purposes. Any woman in this situation needs to detoxify following the various steps covered in the many chapters of this book.

Immune System Breakdown
This is the consequence of the overwhelming of the body's natural self repair system by the various toxins computer use exposes users to, coupled with the lowered production

of natural immune boosting biochemicals due to the deficit in neurotransmitters required to activate and control their production.

Low levels in inhibitors such as melatonin and GABA is a recipe for trouble.

Light sensitivity
This can lead to huge mental problems that will only resolve when the light sensitivity issue is resolved which is a long arduous experience

It can actually result in a loss of life if misdiagnosed and consequently untreated or mistreated. I suffered this and promise you it is real and life threatening.

If you are reading this and believe you may have this issue, please read my books *Lessons I Learned the hard way* and *Eyes, Vision and Computer Use* for more information

Now I will go into how we humans got into all these problems and how we can dig our way out.

Darkness
Darkness from which all objects are made is carbon in its purest form. Thus darkness is the basis for all objects. All elements have three dimensions just like the objects made from them
.

It is this knowledge that helped develop plastic. All we do is look for how to get the carbon particles to bind in a particular chain to produce a certain object by using things like molds.

Science is really easy to understand once you understand the way codes operate and get an understanding of the writings of my ancestors or directly from the code itself as presented in the nature and human machine user manual, which is where my ancestors too got their writing.

I am only continuing the work of my ancestors – being the light..

In this book, I refer to the nature and human machine user manual we call the Bible or Scriptures.

It is the source for all the information presented in my books and not thoughts.

There is no other source of understanding. Even the evil spirits only know what is revealed to we the Jews (once you miss it in understanding who the Jews are, you will have problems with the Scriptures.

Only the real Jews – black people with kinky hair fit exactly with what the Scriptures say about Jews. Only they have the kinky hair, which identifies them as the sheep of God and only they have the pigmentation required to receive the abundance of light fields required to truly receive from God without error.

 That is the reason why they are the only ones the covenant could be made with and they are supposed to spread the light to others.

The manual says it is through us that the information is made public to the whole creature. It says that even angels want to know these things, but that they have to wait for it to be revealed to my people).

I will now delve into the truth and not be politically correct for the sake of us all.

We should tell the truth about who the real Jews are i.e. the black people with kinky hair and encourage them to be themselves instead of trying to dispossess them of their heritage.

The Jews is the light to the Gentiles and is the only source of light to the rest of the world.

The fact that I am writing all these revelations shows that our maker is still pouring out his mercy upon us through the Jew.

Most Jews live in Africa classified as third world having been deceived into giving up their advanced science a long time ago.

New discoveries they make are routinely taken from them under false pretenses and in fact many have been deceived into not knowing who they are and the whole earth is suffering as a consequence as they are not providing the light that only they can provide.

Many in the so called third world lament their so called lack of progress. They do not lack progress as what we are all calling progress is self destruction.

The world has delved into parts of the Hebrew writings given to my ancestors as they studied the Old Testament they were not supposed to, as there parts were not given for operation but as an explanation of what God has done and will do.

Bringing them forth out of greed for wealth is the problem we are all in right now.

We have unleashed things that are not in synch with the rest of nature, are lifeless and are therefore toxic to the rest of nature resulting in things like global warming, cancers and other diseases with no cure, plastic and other materials that cannot biodegrade, clothing and building materials that cannot "breathe" and so on.

Consequently, instead of health that we seek we have death and destruction and are now trying to go back to the old ways and have so messed up the system that now to eat natural food, one must be rich thus consigning people without wealth to a life of misery and destruction.

We do not know our way out of the problem. It is certainly not the various nature destroying experiments we continue to carry out nor the space travels that are the main reason for global warming though no one want to admit this.

The error filled technology age we have unleashed is not compatible with consumption of genetical modified or chemical, pesticide and fertilizer laden food or over dependence on cars rather than walking, or fast foods or chemical laden drugs and so on.

The natural drugs of food grown the way they were intended, the sun, exercise, water and so on is what it is compatible with.

The way out can only be revealed to the real Jews operating as real Jews, which is how I was able to receive the revelations in this book and the others I have written.

I had to go to the God of my fathers as a Jew and ask for revelation as a seed of Abraham, Isaac and Jacob.

Truth is the only way out. Our maker cannot be bribed. The code will run its course and nature must self repair and cast out everything contrary to nature.

The Jews in so called third world countries especially in Africa are indeed better off because their lands have not become totally darkened and they can receive the light to enable the rest of the world come out of the mess it is in.

Instead of trying to be as corrupted as the rest of the world, what they should be doing is acknowledging themselves as Jews, go back directly to the Scriptures, refuse to be defined by the rest of the world and start from the scratch from Genesis.

They should not take anything from anybody. They do not need anyone to affirm them as Jews. The truth of who the real Jews are will be made plain for all to see.

They should refuse the kabala currently being painted as Judaism but should accept the Scriptural Judaism that has Jesus as the High Priest and fully enter into the new covenant through the old. They need to get more into the Old Testament and their history, which is from Genesis to Revelation.

This is the peace of the earth according to the Scriptures. This is the only way the peoples on the earth can receive the knowledge they are looking for of how the human body can live forever. It is available in the Scriptures but only the Jews operating as Jews can receive it.

It is therefore in everybody's interest for the Jews to at last begin to know themselves and stop trying to be from Ham or Japheth.

Noah did not leave anything to Ham so trying to be Ham cannot work because he is diffused into Japheth and Shem. Others trying to deceive the real Jews as is going on today is counterproductive.

Let them be themselves, for the sake of us all.

While I write about the Hebrew writings, I have never seen them. Everything I have written is direct revelation. It just shows the maker's love in that he continues to give Jews revelation so that things not addressed in the writings can be addressed if humans choose to repent from the current path of self destruction.

While everyone need to work on their diet, people of European descent who want to avoid the horrible consequences of computer use over time need to watch their diet more closely and ensure even more so than the pigmented people that it contains the right amino acids, enzymes and so on required for the action of converting the inhibitors in the sunlight to that needed in a moving body like the human machine.

That is because they are unable to receive and retain as much as others. Everyone needs to know their natural limitations and work on them as required.

Chapter 6
The Home/ Work Balance

As discussed in chapters 4 and 5, women generally produce a high level of excitatory neurotransmitters especially during our child bearing age period that prepares us for the job of protecting and caring for the fetus, baby and the born child.

This helps to keep us alert to danger and gives us a heightened capacity to react.

This is a delicate balance as over production of excitatory neurotransmitters means there is a low production of inhibitory ones, which control them.

Computer use uses up a lot of inhibitory neurotransmitters, which can lead to a whole host of issues from the resultant imbalance.

We may for example find it difficult to balance our home/work life resulting in neglect of the children in many cases.

This is also why many of us find it difficult to handle our energetic and active kids resorting to letting them play with computer and computer devices such as ipads and cell phones when we know that as growing children whose brains are still developing, they should not be exposed to the various biochemical and nutrient depletions inherent in computer use.

We just feel overwhelmed and because we are low in inhibitors, we over produce excitatory neurotransmitters such as noradrenalin and use it all up in getting excited and hyper active during computer use.

Then because there are not enough inhibitors such as GABA to initiate new production and help us stay calm, we become depleted in adrenalin and other excitatory biochemicals responsible for enabling us recognize danger and are as a result of all these depletions, unable to make right choices and discern what is not good for us.

We become unable to make the right choices for our children and we become complacent unable to recognize the dangers to our children until they get hurt or the repercussion show up many years down the road.

We may also find ourselves unable to handle criticism indeed unable to understand why no one seems to understand our point of view taking offense because we lack the light fields to enable us understand our faults and cope with them.

We may also find it difficult to understand others or feel empathy even when we think we are doing so.

We may have a delay in being able to analyze thing properly so it may take a long time after an event before we are able to understand it as the analysis will not take place until we have enough biochemical resources to do it by which time we may have reacted wrongly and taken the wrong decision hurting many people.

We will discuss more about this delay in comprehension in the next chapter

We also fall into mood swings from the progesterone/estrogen imbalance that we discussed in chapter 4.

This too affects our familial relationships and many find themselves unable to be patient and end up suing for divorce without thinking things through and only realize they had jumped out too soon after the event or even in some case it may not become clear until many years down the road.

I hope we can see that we really do have a lot of work to do as women if we want to be successful in the technology dependent world we humans have devised.

We cannot therefore live in ignorance. In this instance ignorance is self destruction. The imbalance from computer use will make us procrastinate more than usual, it will make us more emotional, more given to tears.

Weight gain is also a real danger because of the unnatural stress in computer use our bodies are not coded for and which consequently results in more production of cortisol a hormone that is implicated in weight gain.

We may need to reconsider the wisdom of being wired up 24/7.

Computer use should not be a form of leisure. We should only use computers as needed. Computers can never relax us as it cannot stimulate our hearts to stimulate our brains to produce neurotransmitters as it has none to transfer to us.

We receive the neurotransmitters that calm us down from the sun. Going for a long walk instead of staying wired on the Internet or play station is a good idea.

Physically seeing and talking to people is also healthier. The phone should not replace physical contact but complement it. .

Chapter 7
Mental Health

Unbeknown to many people computer use affects the mental capability of all users to varying degrees and the level of hurt is cumulative.

When we hurt, we do not have the resources to see we are hurting as we are depleted in the inhibitors we need for this inherently by computer use

In fact all computer users are schizophrenic to various degrees and procrastinate due to biochemical depletion.

We also become more aware of other people's faults and become more critical unable to see we are just as guilty and become overly focused on others unable to analyze our own selves.

We become unable to handle truth that hurts or even acknowledge truth, as the ability to do this needs light.

All virtues like truthfulness, patience and so on and the ability to truly discern when we run foul of these virtues are dependent on abundance of inhibitors i.e., calming light fields.

Excitatory neurotransmitters make us jump to conclusions and react too soon taking matters into our own hands.

That is why it is dangerous to combine heavy computer use with easy gun access and also why the availability of dangerous information on the Internet has proven a disaster so many times.

The ability to know the difference between right and wrong and to analyze the events around that one sees and hears depends on what is in the database of the heart and the level of the availability of the inhibitors required to correctly analyze the situation or information or image under consideration.

It also depends on the availability of the inhibitors responsible for messaging the activation and control of the various inhibitors and excitatory groups of neurotransmitters required for carrying out the required action.

There is therefore a direct link between the activity of computer use and the continuing state of the mental health of users.

In chapter 9, I discuss the various preventative and management solutions that computer users may need to assist them minimize and manage the inherent mental health in computer use.

The main thing is the need for all to acknowledge that indeed computer use does have a negative cumulative effect on user's neurotransmitter balance which could have a negative effect on women users' hormonal, mental and relational and body organ health.

SAD

The symptoms of seasonal affective disorders (SAD) that afflicts people especially women in the cold months of winter is very similar to what computer users may feel and which could become more pronounce during the winter months and consequently misdiagnosed as SAD.

In addition, because of the natural low intensity of sunlight in this period, computer users may find themselves being more cranky during the winter months i.e. computer use actually exacerbates the symptoms of SAD.

It is important to know that both the number of hours of sun access and the intensity (the heat it produces) are important.

Depression and other behavioral problems

Depression is a result of neurotransmitter imbalance especially a shortfall in the serotonin levels.

Inhibitory neurotransmitters are received from the sun and converted from that operating in a static body to that for a moving one through a complex reaction with amino acids.

The amino acids plus residual undetectable serotonin and other messaging biochemicals responsible for breaking down the food taken to its various components are involved in this conversion process.

As many people stay away from the sun during working hours, it is small wonder that the level of depression among women in countries where people work in such offices and colder countries where there is a natural deficiency in access to sunlight is high.

Attention deficit

The deficiency in inhibitors coupled with over production of excitatory neurotransmitters results in more messaging of action instructions than is required, resulting in attention deficit.

As a consequence, people could become misdiagnosed with ADHD and other attention deficit disorders.

Other behavioral problems that resemble bipolar, autism and so on may be manifested as a result of the high unnatural stress level and the over concentration inherent in computer use.

Schizophrenia
Every computer user is schizophrenic in varying degrees.

That is why we run away from what would help us prevent self damage and instead go for the things that would hurt us.

We would rather take soda than water for example.

We would also prefer to read novels on darkness and violence rather than reading the user manual and many even deny their maker and want to be away from the healing strength of the controls he has put in place to prevent us from self destroying for this same reason.

Procrastination
Many computer users may find themselves procrastinating excessively unable to carry out actions they know they need, rationalizing away things they should not. This is also evidence of depletions in inhibitory neurotransmitters.

Delay in Comprehension
This is a subject many people find difficult to explain to others.

Because of the shortfall in messaging biochemicals it sometimes take a while for computer users to fully understand what they are being told and what they think they are hearing may not be what is being said.

This misunderstanding is a result of a shortfall in the available light fields needed for full comprehension.

Consequently, the brain produces a temporary analysis that can be arrived at with the level of resources it has at that point in time not the analysis it should do.

As soon as it is able to accumulate enough light fields, which may take anywhere from a few minutes to a number of days, it will rewind the incident and correctly analyzes it.

One suddenly just has a flashback to the incidence and has clarity of the questions being posed and what the right answer should have been.

It would seem as if the event is replayed in the head like a rewind and full comprehension takes place after the fact.

This can lead to a lot of quarrels and misunderstandings because the person posing the question may think a deliberate wrong answer was given.

Only someone who has been through it can understand this phenomenon.

Most people do not realize it is due to their computer use and when they do they have no clue as to why computer use is affecting them like that nor what they need to do.

This issue can even be coupled with speech issues so that they say something different from what they think they are saying or are trying to say.

Sometimes their words could come out as gibberish.

The problem is the shortfall in inhibitory neurotransmitters such as GABA used up in the computer use activity without replenishment due to absence of sunlight.

This is coupled with nutrient deficiency as well as dehydration in some cases as many drink soda and other drinks instead of water during computer use.

Nobody eats with computer use in mind. We should as computer use places a lot of demand on certain nutrients especially iron. Please refer back to chapter 2 where we discussed about light.

Excessive Stress

Computer use places excessive stress on the body's system because we are not coded to look directly at a source of light to read.

Our bodies are also coded to exercise most of our body's muscles in concert when carrying out most of life's activities.

Computer use makes us use a few muscles while keeping the others static, leading to friction and stress.

If we are always on the computer for long, without taking breaks to move around and exercise our bodies, that is a recipe for trouble

There is also the issue of weight gain as cortisol is excessively produced. as a result of this stress.

Being immobile for long, while eating junk, which happens a lot for computer user is a recipe for weight gain.

Please refer to my books – *Obesity and Computer Use* , *Computer use induced stress* and *Computer Use Related Health Conditions* for more information on this subject.

Chapter 8
Fibroids, Cancer and body organs malfunction

The hormonal imbalance we discussed in chapter 4 is a recipe for the development of fibroids in women computer users as we discussed in that chapter.

The effect of electromagnetic fields emanating from operating computers could increase the occurrence of cancer especially in women.

What are electromagnetic fields?
As the name suggests electromagnetic fields are naturally magnetized electrical fields.

It is this attribute that results in the formation of objects.

Everything in existence are the results of electrical fields of various combinations, configurations and frequencies that are magnetized to each other in particular concentrations to form solid objects.

Both darkness and light are combinations of electromagnetic fields and the reason we see an object such as a human or a computer is because the object is emitting light out of darkness in various dimensions and combination to make up what we see.

Hence removing electromagnetic fields from computers is an impossibility.

Darkness and light, water and sound are all electromagnetic fields coded and combined in various combinations and frequencies to form them.

Actually, light shines out of darkness. The fields that form light are coded in such a way and intensity to overcome darkness and shine out of it. In fact we see objects such as humans because they emit light out of darkness in various dimensions to form the objects we see them as.

Hence one could call objects solid darkness emitting light in various dimensions and combinations to manifest as objects.

All naturally occurring electromagnetic fields have life. It is life that controls their code.

However life is not electromagnetic fields but is a different dimension that controls and operates in electromagnetic fields.

It can break them down and combine them to form biochemicals such as enzymes, hormones, and neurotransmitters. Artificially generated light is however lifeless.

Life cannot be seen or detected. We only know a person is alive by the activities of their vital sign not that we can detect or test life. We do not and cannot control life. In fact life controls us.

Consequently, it is impossible for us to code life into anything developed by man as we are under its control.

Because artificially generated light is lifeless there is a conflict right down to the cell level in us when we expose ourselves to it.

The closer and the more frequent the exposure the more damage may be done. Hence the root cause of the damaging effect of modern technology.

These issues do not necessarily have to become overwhelming or result in a loss of career. Like the art of using a knife the key is learning how to responsibly take proactive health and lifestyle measures to minimize the negative effects of computer use.

Just as we learned how to use knives without destroying ourselves so we must do with the computer.

Now that we have a better understanding of electromagnetic fields, we can see that the fields of light we call biochemicals responsible for messaging the activity of growth neurotransmitters such as GABA and so on that control and prevent over production of growth hormones, if depleted can result in over firing of growth hormones resulting in fibroids.

Because of the toxicity of the artificial hormones present in computer light and electrical charges that emanate from operating computers as well as the artificial nature of the various elements such as silicon that is use in producing the computer screen can result in cancer.

The nutrient depletions in computer use may make some of the natural solutions for fibroid not feasible most especially because of the effect on iron uptake. For example chamomile, burdock root and so on affect the body's uptake of iron and may not be a good fibroid solution for computer users

Organ malfunction

Various body organs can become affected by the toxic chemicals and minerals women are exposed to in computer use. I, for example came up with various issues including liver cysts and gallstones.

A mineral that is heavily used up in computer use is iron. Consequently child bearing age women that lose a lot of iron as a result of the menstrual cycle can easily become iron deficient with the attendant organ function issues that result from iron deficiency.

Magnesium can also become depleted so that a combination of iron and magnesium deficiency can lead to light sensitivity heart related issues that the medical profession has little understanding of and which cannot be resolved by medication or other conventional medical method. This issue is thoroughly discussed in my first book *Lessons I learned the hard Way* a 300 page guide for computer users.

I urge all to get a copy as I will not be able to give more detailed information in the current book which is supposed to be a short informative book that people can get general information from.

Vitamin C and B as well as many trace minerals are used up heavily in computer use. In fact all the nutrients that the earth and consequently all that is made from it uses in handling the presence of light is use up heavily in computer use.

The big difference is that natural processes are coded into nature and provision is made in the code of our being for replenishment.

Many of us spend most of our days away from the sun, our source of inhibitory neurotransmitters and do not specifically eat for the nutritional demands of computer use.

Consequently we suffer many computer use induced nutrient deficiencies.

Other Issues

Other issues that may arise as a result of computer use include these that I suffered:

1. Severe Nerve infection (including those mimicking Carpel Tunnel Syndrome. It was not carpel Tunnel Syndrome)
2. Nerve ends boil breakouts
3. Ringing ears
4. Constipation/digestive problems
5. Back pain/whole body pain

And so on…

Chapter 9
Dehydration

Many women would find themselves feeling excessively thirst during computer use but may not relate to it as one of the many health consequences of computer use and fail to observe the simple procedures normally used to mange dehydration.

The second issue is that hormonal imbalance is exacerbated by dehydration. Consequently, issues such as the feeling of stress, irritability and so on are compounded resulting in a feeling of being overwhelmed.

It is therefore important to know that dehydration is inherent in computer use. I will explain why.

Just as hydroelectric power uses water to conduct and generate electricity so our skin receptors and eyes need to be hydrated for electrical fields to pass through them to our hearts, brains and so on.

Water is an essential component of our physical structure and in fact the brain has a huge chunk of its composition (over 70%) being water. Indeed the electrical currents that pass through the brain and that produce the energy for its function need water to pass through much like hydro electric power is generated

Water is the medium through which light travels within and into all living beings on earth.

The process of dehydration is one of the final stages of life as dehydration leads to the loss of the electromagnetic elements needed for the flow of messaging biochemical light fields that operate the body

Consequently, the issue of dehydration as a result of computer use is an important factor that affects our brain function and consequently various aspects of our health.

Computer use induced dehydration apart from the water issue also has a toxic chemicals exposure issue as many of the chemicals we are exposed to from the light, cables and materials use in producing the computer are toxic to the human system. For more information on this please refer to my book – *Water, Dehydration and Computer Use*

Many women generally get dehydrated very easily and carry bottles of water with them wherever they go.

Women seem to feel dehydration faster than men or maybe they are not as aware of their bodies and when it hurts as women are.

Just as the light of the sun dehydrates us and we feel thirsty when walking on a sunny day so it is when we are in front of the computer.

Our skin and various receptors in them and the air around us become dehydrated. More so as most of us work in offices without windows or if they have windows they are kept permanently shut.

It is easy for the light emanating from the computer to dehydrated the air it passes through as it comes off the computer screen totally dehydrated and needs to be hydrated to pass through the air unto us

One area I have found that becomes very heavily affected is the skin at the sides of the eyes resulting in dry eyes from the drying of the muscles and the glands responsible for watering our eyes with tears i.e. the tear ducts.

Consequently, the dry eyes many computer users experience is not from the eyes themselves but from the skin an underlying muscles an nerves around the eyeballs.

This is why eye drops do not resolve the issue.

The moisturizers we women apply on our skin before makeup is good but not enough. In addition, they contain several chemicals that may react with the chemicals in the computer monitor light to dehydrate our skin.

Lying on one's back periodically during the day with wet cotton balls placed on the eyelid and washing the face at least twice a day helps in keeping the skin around the eyes hydrated resulting in less dry eyes.

I came across a more effective way in the spraying of PH balanced spring water from which several chemicals and minerals have been removed making close to the water in the earth of the earth and our internal system.

I find the skin is able to absorb that more easily and it is much more effective in reducing dry eyes.

For people who work in offices, this is a big help as it is unlikely one will be able to find anywhere in the office to lie down and do the wet cotton balls option.

I discovered this PH balanced water alternative called "Nature's mist" when the manufacturers Bio Logic Aqua Technologies sent me their products as a complementary gift for being a guest speaker on their talk show – The

Sharon Kleyne Hour – a show dedicated to issues related to the importance of water to the human system.

It was presented as a product to help me in moisturizing my skin to ensure makeup stays in place for longer than usual. I decided to give it a try instead as an aid for reducing dry eyes and found that it worked just fine. It is available on their website http://www.biologicaqua.com/home.php. I strongly recommend it to all computer users.

A second thing to do is to crack open the window and let the fresh air in. These two things complement each other and both need to be in place for maximum benefit. This may be something to discuss with your boss at the next meeting.

Some computer users may find their urine becoming dark and even smelly after long periods of computer us. That is a consequence of dehydration caused by computer use as well as the kidneys being forced to overwork trying to eliminate the toxins that we are exposed to during computer use.

Consequently, my advice is to drink water during computer use to prevent your kidneys from overwork

For more detailed reading on the dehydration angle of things please get hold of my book – *Water, Dehydration and Computer Use*

Chapter 10
Other Suggested Solutions

The artificial light we develop is lifeless and spreads death. The more of it is in anything the more death there will be in that object. If that object is exposed to more of living light, then there is more life. Hence one of the ways to reduce the effect of computer use is to reduce other exposures to lifeless electromagnetic fields in the form of foods, light and so on.

I am advocating some simple solutions including the following. The essence here is to detoxify the body both spiritually and physiologically. All areas are affected and must be treated in a darkness reducing and light increasing way.

Treatment must be all natural to reduce the presence of lifeless artificial light and darkness thereby reducing their presence in such a way that life is more dominant and can cope with the presence of limited lifeless light without being overwhelmed. All the solutions listed are geared to do that. Treatment must in essence be holistic

I will tell you what I have found works but the decision is yours no one can take the decision to self-repair fully for anyone else. Remember the script is cast in stone and things must be done in a particular way.

I will not be politically correct, as that will not help you. I will tell you the truth as I see it. You can receive or reject it. The choice is yours but I will do my part in providing you with information.

1. I have said in this book that I learned from the
    Scriptures hence scripture reading is very important
    even if one does not understand what one is reading.

    A person's religious faith or absence of one is irrelevant
    to the need for more life light to balance the lifeless
    light and consequently the additional darkness one is
    exposing oneself to.

    Many people in prior generation have read the Bible for
    knowledge without being Christians acknowledging
    that that is where they will get the truth from.

    If all one wants from the Scriptures is knowledge about
    human existence that is all the light one will receive.

    It is one of those things one can define as a user of the
    human computer.

    All the creator wants is for one to acknowledge him for
    one's own good so one will not do something self
    destructive. He loves all his creation whether one serves
    him or not.

    The essence is that one is looking for more life light to
    make up for the absence of life in the light we are
    exposing ourselves to and to restore the abundance of
    light life in oneself.

    This light can only be obtained from the word of the
    creator since the script is his word. So read the Bible
    and get life light. The Bible is available for everyone. In
    fact most of today's science has its roots in the
    Scriptures.

If you trace your science to the Hebrew writings, they are based on revelations from the Scriptures.

2   Prayer should be a daily practice. Pray specifically in the name of Jesus. This is the only means the code in us provides.

Anybody can pray in the name of Jesus to receive healing if that is what he or she wants. In fact most professing Christians do just that. They do not serve him but just pray to receive.

 I know many people who are of other faiths who have received the healing they want. They did not convert before they got healed or after.

One will get what one desires. If a person wants salvation he or she will get it. Not everybody will be saved but everyone can be healed. He makes it rain on the good and the bad and provides food, nourishment and life to all.

He is no respecter of persons. He knew we would come to this point and he has provided a way of healing for all.

I know many who also read their Bible because of the benefit of knowledge and healing they get from reading it. It is the user's manual given to us.

That is the only place one will get information. One must however read to understand. Do not interpret or else you will get confused. If at first you do not understand continue reading until you do, take one day at a time.

It may take a long time before you begin to understand but you will be getting life light every time you read whether you understand or not.

If you do not stop reading, the time will come when you will begin to slowly understand. At first things will be gray but go on the real understanding will come.

3   Have your doctor do a whole body chemistry analysis of the blood, urine and fecal waste.

The result will not show everything as these tests usually tests for total mineral presence rather than the ionic mineral form needed for nerve messaging but it is a good starting point in identifying what is being depleted and need to be replaced

4.   Physiological Detoxification – juice fasting. This should only be done under the monitoring supervision of a doctor.

5.   Daily sunlight exposure even in winter, Vitamin D is not the only thing you get from the sun It is not even necessarily the most important as we are limited in our knowledge.

 In fact many of life's functions messages are coded in us through the sunlight. You also need the sunlight for neurotransmitters especially brain GABA that can only be produced in the brain, serotonin, Dopamine etc. It seems all biochemicals need sunlight to some extent for production.

That is the code because neurotransmitters are the messaging biochemicals they need a lot of light life, which is coded into us from the sun.

When you exercise outside you get the life light fields from the sun in 2 ways. Directly from the sun and in the air and so we feel recharged and happy and the stress goes down. Taking vitamin D alone will not achieve all of this.

6. Eat Organic – avoid toxins from pesticides etc.

7. Read with the light of the sun daily

8. Going for daily walks where there is greenery and flowers i.e. plenty of bright colors also where there is movement so walk to the park along the road if possible.

    Daily walks are doubly important in the winter months when sunlight is reduced in both intensity and duration resulting in less production of neurotransmitters by the body.

    This is probably why animals hibernate in winter. This natural neurotransmitter production reduction is what leads to seasonal affective disorder and computer users may find themselves prone to this and more incidences of heart and respiratory issues if they fail to go for daily walks.

9. Eat fruits and vegetable. We were created to receive our nutrients and medication from fruits, vegetables and herbs. The combination of fruit and vegetable eaten is important.

10. Eat animal protein from non man adulterated sources only e.g. organic grass fed bison/buffalo, game etc.

11. Exercise. Some outside if possible. Do pure exercises only not meditation. Make things simple. This is no time for experimentation. Look in the Scriptures.

    Anything not there to satisfy our spiritual relationship with our maker do not do it. There is only one way just as with a computer only what is programmed in works.

    Other things may seem to work initially but in the long run will unravel. It may sometimes take a long time for us to realize things are unraveling and may sometimes be too late to undo. It may become a permanent damage.

12. Drink water when thirsty to avoid dehydration

13. Wash the face after computer use

14. Spray Nature's Mist, the PH and composition balanced water we learned about in chapter 8 on face regularly to reduce dry eyes. The PH and composition of atmospheric and the depth of the earth's crust water is different from that of tap water.

15. Get an air purifier with ionization properties. This will increase negative ionization.

16. Make ergonomic changes to your workstation arrangement.

17. Crack open the window for fresh air when using the computer.

18. Make one day in a week a computer free day. In addition take computer free vacations

19. Take many breaks. Take your eyes of the computer every 30 minutes.

20. Have an annual eye examination done. And test for light sensitivity.

21. Vitamin, Mineral and Biochemical such as GABA, Melatonin etc. Supplementation under the advise of your doctor.

22. Establish and maintain healthy relationships with family and friends. We were not created to be self-sustaining. We are all linked in this massive human and earth bound computer network and our actions affect each other even when we cannot see how.

23. If you already have many behavioral issues going on I will advise you to avoid arguments. Walk away, talk to people especially family and friends.

24. Do not isolate yourself as that could have very devastating consequence. Find someone you can talk to before taking decisions as your decision-making ability has probably become impaired even if you are unaware of it.

25. Music – specifically gospel music that are scripturally based.

If you find multivitamins a problem do not worry, that happened to me. What it means is that there is an imbalance that is being exacerbated by the combination of the multivitamin composite.

In my case I had such a bad depletion of iron, magnesium etc. that anything that had calcium in the mix was a problem since calcium reduces the body's ability to uptake iron. In fact I was unable to eat vegetables like broccoli that are rich in calcium for over a year.

I therefore had to stop all vitamins and substituted with diet and supplementing the actual minerals and vitamins depleted.

Hence I had to take magnesium, iron, vitamin B, and so forth supplements. For a while there were so many tablets, capsules and liquids to take with my food daily.

After 1 year I was gradually able to start eating broccoli and so forth and after 3 years of working on this issue, I was fully able to handle multivitamins and I did not have to take iron tablets anymore as long as I eat iron rich foods that do not contain herbicides, chemicals and pesticides.

The best of such foods I have found is organic grass fed bison/buffalo. Your issue may be different. Learning to listen to your body and identifying the issues involved under the supervision of your doctor is what you need to do.

Note:
Sometimes when we take supplements to address some issues e.g. Melatonin, Magnesium and it seems the issue has been arrested, we do not realize it is a warning sign as what we have addressed may not be the only thing wrong.

When the symptoms seem to be under control and we do not change our ways and length of exposure, then warnings cease and after some time that could go into years the crash comes in phased leaps and bounds.

The full effect will result in a major breakdown which at that point may not be identified as being related to computer use but to other issues that have arisen over time that were actually related to computer use but which may be ascribed to other things.

The final breakdown may be misdiagnosed.

For additional or more comprehensive suggested solution please refer to the book *Lessons I Learned the Hard Way*.

Start taking preventive measures today, and see how your health improves. When you take preventive measures, your risk of getting a major breakdown is reduced.

In addition, your healthcare cost will be reduced, your productivity at work will go up and that promotion will become achievable. It also means a better quality of life.

Make the computer a tool that is both a short and a log term blessing and not one that is short-term blessing and long-term curse. The choice is yours to make.

Like the user manual we call the Bible or Scripture says 'choose life that you may live"

Note to Doctors - Supplementation

It is very important to work with medical professionals.

Because of the various depletion of nutrients that occur in computer use addiction, it is important to get complete whole body chemistry analyzing the blood, urine and stool at the minimum to determine as much as possible what has been depleted in order to determine the best nutritional diet to embark upon and to determine if supplementation is necessary.

This analysis does not reveal everything but it is a very important starting point. It should be repeated as needed to track progress and determine necessary changes required in the treatment program.

In addition there will more often than not be a need for GABA and melatonin supplementation. Another thing I will recommend a doctor using is Rhodolia Rosea.

There are other issues such as magnesium, zinc, iron, Vitamin D, B, C and other mineral and vitamin supplementation, but in order to ensure people go to their doctors, I will only go this far. I invite doctors to get in touch with me via the email address provided in "Note to the reader" for more information on supplementation. You can also read my book *Lessons I Learned the Hard way*.

Computer use induced health conditions should never be self diagnosed and treated without medical help to monitor the process. It is very dangerous to try to do it on your own. Get your doctor my books and get him or her to contact me for things like checklists, supplementation and other matters I consider too risky to provide to the general public.

Note To The Reader:

About the author:

Adetutu Ijose, is a technology and accounting professional with over 25 years of intensive computer use exposure who suffered life threatening computer related health conditions the doctors could neither diagnose not treat.

In desperation and with a good knowledge of codes and how they work, she studied the human computer user manual we call the Bible until she was able to understand why and how the computer hurts our body's system as well as the preventive and repair kits placed in nature by our maker.

She also began to realize that many issues not normally attributable to computer use were actually due to or exacerbated by computer use.

Being a woman she also discovered there were some unique gender issues too

Adetutu Ijose seeks in this book to bring this fact to every woman's attention in a bid to help computer users achieve and maintain a goo quality of life since computers are here to stay and are indispensable in today's world.

Because our modern lifestyle of heavy computer use is not going to change anytime soon, she realized that it was important to make the information she had public in a bid to help everyone.

She is now passing on her understanding about computer use induced issues through her many books, other writings and speaking activities so others can receive help.

Adetutu Ijose is a speaker on the subject of computer use induced health conditions. She is also a contributor to several online article websites and blogs including content sites Yahoo Contributor Network and examiner.com. She has also been interviewed on radio. She in addition became ordained as an Evangelist in 2008.

To schedule a speaking or consulting engagement, interview, so on with the author, please contact Adetutu Ijose at http://www.foodsthathealdaily.com.

For Adetutu Ijose's online press kit or for press releases and other media matters and inquiries, please go to http://lessosilearnedthehardway.com/AdetutuIjoseMediaPressKit.aspx

Discover other titles by Adetutu Ijose to help you better understand responsible computer use and how computer use affect us all as well as what we need to do to prevent and manage these issues at www.foodsthathealydaily.com, www.amazon.com and other online stores. Ebook versions of this and other books by Adetutu Ijose are available at amazon.com, Barnes and Nobles, Smashword.com and other ebook stores. A complete list is provided below.

Email Adetutu Ijose at adetutuijose@gmail.com or computerblessings@gmail.com

Connect with Adetutu Ijose Online:
Facebook: http://www.facebook.com/home.php

Read Adetutu Ijose's blogs at
http://lessonsilearnedthehardway.blogspot.com/ and
http://adetutuijose.wordpress.com/ and
http://www.foodsthathealdaily.com/Pages/Articlesandblogs.aspx

Computer Use Induced Health Conditions related books by Adetutu Ijose as at the time of writing are:

1) *Lessons I Learned the Hard Way: How to Identify, Minimize, Treat and Manage Computer Related Health Condition*

2) *Computer Related Health Condition: Understanding the Human Computer*

3) *Healing Juicing Smoothie and Milk Shake Recipes: Juices, Smoothies and Milk Shakes that Help the Body Achieve its Self Healing Process*

4) *Healing Meals Recipe: Meals that Help the Body Achieve its Self Healing Process*

5) *Cyber Bullying: How and Why Bullies operate*

6) *Global Epidemic: The Human Abuse of the Computer*

7) *Computer Use Addiction and Withdrawal Syndromes: What You Need to Know*

8) *Teenage and Adult Texting Addictions: What You Need to Know*

9) *Allergies, Asthma and Computer Use: The Contributory Effects of Computer Use to Allergies and Asthma Trends*

10) *Computer Use Induced Stress: What You Need to Know*

11) *The Health effect of Video Games: What You Need to Know*

12) *Eyes, Vision and Computer Use: How You can Protect Yourself From Technology Use Induced Harm*

13) *Obesity and Computer Use: What You Need to Know*

14) *Water, Dehydration and Computer Use: Learn How to Protect Yourself*

15) *The Health Effect of Computer Use on Women: What Every Woman Needs to Know*

For other titles published after this book –*The Health Effects of Computer Use on Women*, please go to amazon.com and other online stores or visit my website www.foodsthathealdaily.com Ebook versions are also available for kindle, ipad, kobo, sony, nook, smashwords.com and other ebook readers

INDEX

A

Activities, 16, 18, 31, 40, 42, 61, 64, 67, 85
Artificial, 9, 18, 19, 26, 29, 30, 31, 40, 67, 68, 75

B

Balance, 16, 29, 30, 36, 42, 47, 48, 56, 60, 76
Bible, 5, 13, 21, 31, 40, 51, 76, 77, 83, 85
Biochemical, 11, 20, 27, 32, 57, 59, 71, 81
Biochemicals, 15, 16, 17, 18, 25, 29, 31, 50, 57, 61, 63, 67, 68, 78
Body, 6, 9, 13, 15, 16, 17, 18, 19, 24, 29, 30, 35, 37, 38, 54, 55, 60, 61, 66, 69, 70, 71, 75, 78, 79, 84, 87,
Book, 5, 6, 12, 19, 21, 23, 24, 27, 28, 31, 32, 37, 42, 43, 49, 51, 53, 69, 72, 74, 76, 83, 84, 85, 88
Brain, 40, 63, 71, 72, 78

C

Chemicals, 17, 29, 30, 69, 72, 73, 82
Children, 26, 27, 28, 39, 47, 56, 57, 61
Choice, 42, 52, 54, 55, 56, 92, 101
Choices, 34, 43, 44, 45, 46, 75
Code, 5, 10, 12, 14, 15, 16, 21, 22, 23, 31, 33, 35, 36, 38, 42, 44, 46, 50, 54, 58, 67, 69, 77, 78,
Coded, 9, 10, 11, 17, 18, 22, 33, 34, 38, 42, 64, 66, 67, 69, 78
Computer, 5, 6, 8, 9, 10, 11, 12, 16, 18, 19, 20, 21, 24, 25, 26, 29, 30, 31, 32, 35, 40, 41, 42, 46, 48, 49, 50, 55, 56, 58, 59, 60, 61, 62, 63, 64, 65, 66, 68, 69, 70, 71, 72, 73, 74, 75, 76, 79, 80, 81, 83, 84, 85, 86, 87, 88,

D

Darkness, 13 14, 15, 22, 23, 24, 34, 35, 40, 44, 45, 46, 50, 62, 66, 67, 75, 76
Day, 8, 13, 14, 22, 31, 44, 72, 73, 77, 80
Deficiency, 20, 62, 64, 69
Dehydration, 64, 71,72, 74, 80, 88
Depleted, 6, 25, 37, 38, 39, 59,61, 68, 69, 82, 84
Depletion, 27, 31, 36, 41, 48, 56, 59, 81, 84
Depletions, 31, 32, 40, 57, 63, 68
Depression, 24, 29, 48, 61, 62
Diagnose, 6, 8, 20, 21, 85
Diet, 19, 41, 55, 82, 84
Dimensions, 13, 16, 18, 50, 66, 67

E

Earth, 6, 13, 14, 17, 22, 34, 37, 44, 48, 52, 54, 69, 71, 73, 81,
Electromagnetic, 17, 18, 66, 67, 68, 71, 75
Environment, 6, 8, 13, 14, 29, 39, 43
Estrogen, 17, 29, 30 31, 57
Excitatory, 31, 51, 57, 58, 59, 60, 62,
Exercise, 19, 31, 41, 53, 64, 65, 79, 80

F

Female, 29, 33, 37, 47
Fundamental, 34, 35,37, 38, 44

G

GABA, 17, 41, 48, 50, 57, 64, 68, 78, 81, 84
Grace, 34, 42, 43, 44, 45

H

Health, 5, 6, 9, 11,20, 21, 29, 29, 48, 53, 59, 60, 65, 68, 71, 83, 84, 85, 86, 87, 88

S

Science, 5, 10, 17, 50, 52, 76, 77
Scriptures, 5, 17, 21, 42, 51, 54, 76, 77, 80
Serotonin, 17, 31, 61, 78
Sex, 26, 32, 33, 38
Sexual, 33, 34, 35, 37, 38, 42, 44
Solution, 5, 20, 30, 39, 83
Solutions, 6, 19, 20, 60, 68, 75
Soul, 13,15, 16, 17, 28, 37, 38
Sun, 6, 17, 18, 19, 26, 31, 41, 53, 58, 61, 62, 70, 72, 78, 79
System, 5, 6, 17, 18, 19, 22, 27, 29, 30, 33, 37, 41, 49, 53,
    64, 72, 73, 74, 85

T

Technology, 19, 46, 53, 58, 68, 85, 88
Toxic, 18,19, 29, 30, 53. 69, 72
Ttoxins, 30, 49, 74, 79
Truth, 10, 20, 25, 33, 41, 42, 43, 46, 51, 52, 54, 59, 75, 76,

U

User manual, 5, 13, 15, 16, 20, 27, 38, 51, 62, 83, 85

V

Video Games, 8, 25, 27, 28, 87
Vitamin, 69, 78, 79, 81, 82, 84

W

Water, 22, 53, 62, 64, 66, 71,72,73.74, 80, 88
Woman, 5, 25, 32, 49, 85, 88
Women, 5, 9, 10, 12, 20, 24, 25 ,27, 28, 29, 30, 32, 38, 42,
    47, 48, 49, 56, 58, 60, 62, 66, 69, 71, 72, 73, 88
Words, 16, 18, 21, 24, 25, 36, 37, 40, 64
Works, 15, 22, 75, 80
World, 8, 9, 11, 24, 25, 30, 32, 35, 52, 54, 58, 85

www.ingramcontent.com/pod-product-compliance
Lightning Source LLC
Chambersburg PA
CBHW070553290526
45790CB00002B/665